SELMA BLAIR

Copyright © 2022
University Press
All Rights Reserved

Table of Contents

Introduction
Chapter 1: Early Life
Chapter 2: New York
Chapter 3: Early Breaks
Chapter 4: Break Out
Chapter 5: Legally Blonde
Chapter 6: Hellboy
Chapter 7: Successful Career
Chapter 8: Personal Life
Chapter 9: Multiple Sclerosis
Chapter 10: A Cathartic Memoir
Conclusion

Introduction

Though never as famous as many other actresses from the 1990s and early 2000s, Selma Blair was an easily recognizable young actress during this time. She had more prominent roles in two teen dramas, one of the naïve teens in Cruel Intentions and the villain in the popular Legally Blonde. She continued to gain a different kind of fanbase when she starred as the love interest in the two Hellboy movies. She continued to stay busy, acting in several indie films through the beginning of the 2010s. Soon, she moved more into TV roles, though she still works in some films.

Her diverse abilities on-screen seem to be more reflective of the significant highs and lows of her life. Blair had admitted in interviews that she started drinking alcohol when she was only five years old and first got drunk when she was around seven years old. After passing out because of drinking alcohol while she was with her 4-year-old son, she decided to finally give up alcohol for good, something she had been unsuccessful at for years. However, she has also said that she thinks the only reason she could make it through her childhood was because of alcohol. Having experienced sexual assault on several occasions and being taken advantage of by a teacher whom she trusted, Blair has long hinted at darker moments in her life that resulted in her contemplating suicide. Alcohol kept her in a state where she felt she could cope with her problems.

Her life changed again in 2018 when she was diagnosed with multiple sclerosis, also known as MS. She has been very open and honest about her experience with the disease, even showing some of her worst days when going through treatment. As horrific as she felt the diagnosis was, it finally provided an answer to the slew of minor health problems she was having during that time. Instead of tackling the symptoms that resulted from the illness, she was able to seek treatment that helped alleviate much of the problem. MS cannot be cured, but treatments can allow sufferers to live more normal lives. During an interview in early 2022, she said that her MS was in remission, so she could live with less pain while being more active. Because she has loved horseback riding since she was 17 years old and enjoys ice skating, being able to do these activities has helped her reach a better state mentally.

Blair has become a much more vocal advocate as she has opened up about her numerous struggles. She has long been less open about the sexual abuse she experienced, but she has been open about her MS and alcoholism. In February 2022, she reported that her now ex-boyfriend attacked her, resulting in her going to the hospital. She was granted a restraining order against him. She had been working on a book of memoirs called *Mean Baby: A Memoir of Growing Up* that was scheduled to come out in May 2022. In the book, she opened up about the sexual abuse she suffered when she was young and said it was the first time she had shared the stories of the experiences. When asked about how she feels today after all of the dark moments covered in the book, she has been incredibly optimistic about her future, saying she is finally in a good place.

Chapter 1

Early Life

Born in Southfield, Michigan, on June 23, 1972, Selma Blair Beitner was the youngest of the four daughters of Elliot and Molly Ann Beitner. Her parents worked in law, with her father being a labor arbitrator and her mother becoming a judge. Outside of her book of memoirs, not much has been discussed about her early life. Her family was Jewish, so she was raised outside of the Christian religion prevalent in the area. She had said that she started drinking when she was five and was an alcoholic by the time she was seven.

During interviews, Blair has said that she always knew that her mother was incredibly difficult and critical, but not without good reason. Her mother had overcome much prejudice to become a judge during a time when men openly discriminated against women. This tough attitude translated into tough love, which created a somewhat complicated relationship between mother and her third daughter. It was only decades later, when her son told her that she was critical, that Blair realized just how much she took after her mother. It helps her better understand the tough love that she received growing up. As Blair pointed out, her mother would not lie about faults and problems but gave it to her daughters straight.

Blair attended Hillel Day School and Cranbrook School. During this time, she had a mentor she has said violated her trust. It was clear that he did not rape her. However, Blair pointed out that the way he allowed his hand to slide down her back while hugging her and then kissing her on the mouth did significant emotional harm to her. She had seen him as a mentor and friend. After the incident, she no longer felt safe because of how uncomfortable and inappropriate his alleged actions were. Like most girls and women who were harassed at this time, she was not sure whom to talk to about the incident. Finally, she decided to tell her mother. Unfortunately, her mother's response was entirely predictable for the time. Blair's mother told her not to tell anyone else. As a result, nothing was done while her mentor continued working at the school. It was a small consolation, but when Blair received an award at the end of her schooling, he turned to congratulate her. Speaking to her mother, he said something along the lines of "You must be so proud." Her mother simply told him, "I know what you did. Stay away from my daughter." It did not really help Blair, but it showed that her mother did believe her.

When Blair made her allegations three and a half decades later, the response was much different. The school let the alumni know that they should contact the school if they have similar stories about misconduct. Unfortunately, the police in the area provided a significantly less helpful response, issuing a statement saying, "If the victim wants to come forward and file a complaint, she's more than welcome to do so. But we don't chase down everything we've heard in a book or article."

The problem is that it is far harder to prove sexual misconduct than most other crimes. For victims, regardless of their gender, having their support system believe them and stick up for them can help. What Blair's mother did was far from what should have happened, but as a judge, she likely knew that it would be all but impossible to do anything against a man who held a high position. While unable to do anything legally, she ensured that the man knew that his misconduct had not gone unreported and that his victim was not entirely alone.

Leaving a very troubled childhood behind, Blair struck out to make her own way in college. But unfortunately, many of the problems she had faced went with her, especially her dependence on alcohol.

Chapter 2

New York

After her high school graduation, Blair applied for and was accepted to Kalamazoo College, a college not too far from home. At least she was still in the same state. She did not seem interested in going into law like her parents, opting to focus on photography and literature. She also had an interest in psychology, and instead of choosing a single field, Blair worked toward two degrees. During a later interview, she said she did not limit her career path, except "I wanted to be a ballerina, a horse trainer, and then I wanted to be a photographer….I just never thought it was feasible for a girl from Michigan to ever make it to the stage or screen and tell a story." That did not mean that she was not interested in acting, pointing to Sissy Spacek as an example of an actress that she looked up to. Blair did not feel that she had the right background to make a career in the field.

Though she had decided it was not the right job for her, it indicated that she had once considered it as a possibility. Moreover, when people think about a job and dismiss it, at some point, they usually revisit the idea, especially when they are young. One of her earliest roles was in *Murder in the Cathedral*, by T.S. Eliot, when she was still in high school. Perhaps one of the reasons she figured acting was not going to be her future was that Blair admitted that she considered her turn in the play a failure. However, one of her teachers had seen her potential and told her to keep trying. While in college, she would listen and make another attempt, this time in a role in the short play *The Little Theater of the Green Goose* by Konstantly Ildefons Galczynski. This experience in college seemed to have been entirely different as Blair's interest in acting and belief that it could actually work for her changed by the time she graduated. She did continue with her education, earning a double major in English and Psychology at the University of Michigan. However, she did not put either of these degrees to use when she decided to find out if she could succeed in acting.

Around this time, her parents had divorced, resulting in Blair dropping her father's last name, Beitner. Instead, she would come to be known by her mother's name, indicating how even their complex relationship was still strong. This was further highlighted when her mother supported her daughter's decision to pursue acting. Not long after graduation, Blair started getting ready to move to the city she thought would be best for an acting career, New York City. When her mother found out, Blair would later recount her reaction, "[she] helped me pack my suitcase, and I moved to New York about a week later."

This proved to be a challenging move, with problems that she may not have entirely anticipated. Alternatively, at least elements she had not really considered. Even though she did not have the funds to live in one of the most expensive cities in the US, Blair seemed to be putting all of her efforts into her career. She ended up at The Salvation Army, a homeless shelter, during her time in the city. Despite not having enough money to live in her own place, she did buy a Versace dress, ensuring that she could attract the eyes of people who might be interested in hiring her for roles. She later recounted that the piece was a comfortable red velvet minidress. She was 21 at the time and talked about how she saved for the dress, focusing on getting the dress and overpaying for a place to live.

She did not move to New York without some idea of what she needed to do. While she did not take care of her lodgings, the hopeful actress enrolled in numerous acting schools, including the Stella Adler Conservatory and Stonestreet Screen Acting Workshops. All of this would start to pay off with minor roles as she looked for her first big break.

Chapter 3

Early Breaks

Having arrived in the Big Apple in 1995, it took her a while to get discovered. She had appeared in a commercial after having gone through about 75 auditions. She also joined the Screen Actors Guild. Though it took a while, she made her first debut on the small screen on a Nickelodeon show called *The Adventures of Pete & Pete*, in the episode "Das Bus." She filled a guest role on the show. In 1996, she would make her debut on the big screen in the movie called *The Broccoli Theory*, and her role was called the Pretzel Cart Lesbian. She also starred in the Canadian movie *Kids in the Hall: Brain Candy*. The *Kids in the Hall* were a popular sketch comedy troupe on Comedy Central in the US. There was some controversy in the movie, as was common for much of what the troupe did. This did help her to gain more attention, and she was soon hired to work on the new sketch comedy called *The Dana Carvey Show*. The show was developed for one of the biggest stars to leave Saturday

Night Live in the 1990s, Dana Carvey. Many people were planning to watch because they were excited to see what the funny actor would do with his own show. The show did not perform well because critics saw it as controversial and offensive after the first show. However, several future big names were on the show, including Stephen Colbert. Blair's role was uncredited, so the show's cancellation did not affect her much.

Though she continued to get minor roles, Blair did appear in increasingly more prominent films. First, she had a role in the highly anticipated movie *In & Out*, which starred Kevin Cline. She then took the lead role in the movie *Strong Island Boys*, playing Tara. She won one role in *Scream 2*, though her part was just as a friend on the phone to Sarah Michelle Gellar's character, Cici.

While she was able to stay busy with more minor roles, much of this time was more prominently defined by two roles that she almost won that would have jump-started her career a year or two before her major breakout role. Both of the roles were TV roles, but they were in shows that would be major successes, jump-starting the careers of most of the major actors in the shows. The first show where she was almost cast as the primary female actress was in *Dawson's Creek*. The role of Joey went to Katie Holmes, who went on to be best known for marrying the much older actor Tom Cruise. Though she did continue to act, Holmes's career was far less high profile after her marriage to the megastar, particularly after the way he announced they were dating and expressed how much he loved being around her. Holmes most notable role was as Rachel Dawes in *Batman Begins*. She was replaced in the second movie, The *Dark Knight Rises*, by Maggie Gyllenhaal. Though there was speculation as to why she did not return for the role, it has since been reported that Holmes was more interested in branching out into other areas. Had she known how beloved the second film was, and it has been considered the best in the trilogy, some people find it hard to believe that she willingly left the franchise. However, she could not have known how much the audience would love the role, especially as the casting of Heath Ledger as the Joker was met with a lot of scorn and criticism. Holmes did remain busy until her marriage, and she continues to act occasionally, usually in minor roles. Since her divorce, she has been more active in film, though she has still largely remained out of the limelight.

The second role that Blair almost got remains a top-rated show today, *Buffy the Vampire Slayer*. She had auditioned for the role of Buffy. Ironically, she lost that role to Sarah Michelle Gellar. Not only would she be a voice actor on the phone with Gellar in *Scream 2*, but Blair would also go on to be in a major film with Gellar not long after Buffy became incredibly popular. Gellar would be incredibly active in the industry, becoming one of the most popular scream queens in the horror genre. She had initially auditioned for the role of Cordelia in *Buffy* and instead was cast as Buffy. Gellar would be cast in roles more similar to Cordelia in films. Besides being the first major character killed off in *Scream 2* (in a role similar to Drew Barrymore's in *Scream*), Gellar played Helen Shivers in the movie *I Know What You Did Last Summer*. Since her character was killed off, she did not return in the sequel. She also played the lead role in the horror movie *The Grudge*, a remake of the Japanese horror movie, *Ju-On*. This was one role where she was the final girl, but she was quickly killed off in the next movie. Gellar also went on to play Daphne in the *Scooby Doo* movies. She went on to marry her co-star from those films, Freddie Prince Jr., though they actually met on the set of *I Know What You Did Last Summer*. She was an incredibly popular actor for years after *Buffy* ended. She continued to act in TV, movies, and video games, though she shifted focus after having children. While she does still appear on screen from time to time, Gellar has been more active on social media, writing cookbooks, and supporting charities.

Selma missed out on these career-defining roles that would have significantly opened the door for her acting career. While she would not have the same kind of success as the two women who did get the roles, Blair would be far more successful than she had thought possible. She would not burst onto the scene the same way, but she would manage to have a reasonably stable career and earn a place in several fandoms over several decades. Blair seemed to have a really good relationship with both women. Years later, she would post a picture of her with both ladies with the caption, "in honor of #creek week and all things new again, I have always admired these ladies. Even if I did not get the part of #joey potter. The role was all @katieholmes212, and I loved watching her from the start. I auditioned for #Buffy but did not even come close. But I have a friend for life. Love you @sarahmgellar this was the night we won #bestkiss #mtv movie awards 2000." This referenced her first major role in which she and Gellar worked together on screen.

Chapter 4

Break Out

Blair managed to keep an optimistic outlook after losing two significant roles. This might have been easier to do, considering she seemed to stay pretty active with her own roles. However, all of her work would come to fruition in 1999 when she was cast in two movies that would be considered teenage genre-defining films for the 1990s. She would take on two very different roles in the films, which likely helped her avoid the stereotyping that most other actors face. When she did start to gain recognition, it was as much because of how versatile she was on screen.

Her first major role was in the movie *Cruel Intentions*, released in 1999. Blair played Cecile Caldwell, a young teenager whose parents had just moved to New York City. The family does not quite fit into the wealthy families considered "old money," so they spend less time paying attention to their daughter. The character was incredibly naïve and childish, but the fact that she was inexperienced seemed to be the primary draw for Court Reynolds. When Cecile started at the new school with Court, Kathryn Merteuil, and Sebastian Valmont, Court and the more knowledgeable and experienced Kathryn were a couple. After meeting the inexperienced Cecile, he dumped Kathryn, saying he was in love with the new girl. Angry and looking for revenge, Kathryn gets her step-brother Sebastian to seduce Cecile, ruining her for Court. Kathryn plays a prominent role in the successful plan as she initially befriended the girl who unwittingly stole Kathryn's boyfriend. Kathryn helped to guide her into Sebastian's arms. As a young teen who had no experience in the big city, Cecile looked up to Kathryn and was willing to listen to the malicious advice, not realizing what was happening. The role was a large one for Blair, though she was not one of the three major players in the film.

The movie included one of the first on-screen kisses between two women, Gellar and Blair. It even won them an award, which Blair mentioned about 35 years later in her post. She enjoyed her time with the stars Gellar, Ryan Phillippe (who played Sebastian Valmont), and Reese Witherspoon (who played Annette Hargrove, a much more arduous sexual conquest for Sebastian).

The role was a unique challenge for several reasons. There was an age gap between Blair and the character, which was not as evident in the movie. Given Blair's life experiences, her personality was vastly different from the fairly cringey young teen that she played. Though the character came off as annoying, Blair's portrayal differed from the other characters because she was younger than the other teens (she was a freshman, while the rest were at the end of their high school careers). She also came from a less exclusive place than the other teens, making her stand out and seem pretty clueless about most things. The character did stand out as more annoying, particularly compared to the older teenager Annette. Annette intentionally abstained from sex because she had formed ideas about sex (having reached an age where teens generally felt more pressure).

The plot was a retelling of the film *Dangerous Liaisons*, released in 1988 and starring Glenn Close (Kathryn's adult counterpart), John Malkovich (Sebastian's adult counterpart), and Michelle Pfeiffer (Annette's adult counterpart). It was considered a much darker teen drama than most other movies being produced at the time.

Many of the plot points and actions of the main characters would be considered criminal today. It was the early days of the Internet, so laws had not been made against some of the activities the teens committed online. Considering the age of Cecile compared to the others, some have brought up the problem with her seduction; Annette is roughly the same age, so her seduction is not viewed in the same way. Alcohol is also used during Cecile's seduction, which is viewed in much harsher terms today as that behavior has been re-examined following the *Me Too Movement*. While some say that the film would not be acceptable today, it could be argued that the horrible actions and unethical behavior were precisely the movie's point. Not everything that Kathryn and Sebastian do is illegal, but other things are, including blackmail. Like in *Dangerous Liaisons*, that highlighted just how horrible the two step-siblings are. If there is a problem with the film, it is that Sebastian is treated like a hero at the end because he saves Annette's life, dying in the process. There was no build-up to showing him change or become a decent person. He only returns to her after Kathryn gets angry at him for falling for Annette.

He successfully seduced Annette, then, to make Kathryn happy, he told Annette that he no longer loved her. The character did horrible things, and he did not atone for what he did wrong. Had he not died, perhaps he would have, but the fact that he was treated like a hero after all of the damage he did could be seen as problematic. A lot more growth would be needed today to see him as anything other than a villain who might change.

Whatever the film's legacy, Blair was recognized for her acting abilities, getting her more attention from other producers and directors. This would result in her being considered for an even bigger role in her next big project.

Chapter 5

Legally Blonde

Between 1999 and 2001, Blair had a few roles, but the next big project came with a much bigger role – she played the antagonist in *Legally Blonde*. Her character was the antithesis of her role in *Cruel Intentions*. This extreme difference in characters would help sell her as a more diverse actress than many other women and men her age, which remains incredibly difficult today.

The movie is about Elle Woods (played by Reese Witherspoon), a young woman who goes to dinner expecting her boyfriend, Warner Huntington III (played by Matthew Davis), to propose. He is preparing to go to Harvard Law School, and he does not see her as the kind of woman who will complement his political ambition. To win him back, Wood studies hard, earning a high score on the LSAT. Coupled with her 4.0 GPA, the score earns her an acceptance letter from Harvard Law School. Since she was raised in Southern California, she has an entirely different outlook compared to her predominantly east coast classmates, who do not take her seriously at first. When she finally finds her former boyfriend, Elle learns that he has gotten engaged to one of his exes, Vivian Kensington (played by Blair). Vivian quickly belittles Elles, saying that she is a fool, something that Elle will realize by the end of the film, but for a different reason. Warner again insults Elle, saying she is not smart enough to succeed. Upset by the way she is treated, Elle focuses on doing well. All three of them are chosen to serve as interns to one of the professors in a high-profile case. Elle befriends the client, who is the defendant in a murder trial. When Elle promises not to disclose the client's alibi, the client starts to become more open. Vivian is impressed by Elle's abilities, eventually telling Elle that Warren was only at Harvard because of his dad. With money, Warren would not have been accepted to the school, causing Elle to rethink her opinion of him. Elle eventually helps to catch the actual murderer out on the stand, using her knowledge of fashion and hair products to bring down the murderer. Warren tries to reconnect with Elle after the trial, saying she has proved herself. However, she rejects him, and Vivian dumps him. Over time, Elle and Vivian become good friends, and Elle is asked to give the speech when she graduates a couple of years later.

Blair played the role from several different angles, going first from the woman who jealously protects her relationship with her boyfriend to a more open-minded person. Most of her knowledge about Elle likely came from Warren, leading Blair to play the character from a more protective place who does not understand Elle because of what she has been told. Over time, she gets to know Elle, and the audience sees her character change over the movie. It was one of the few movies that showed women realizing that a man who plays them against each other is not worth it, earning it a lot of attention for the more positive message for young women. The reception was mixed among critics, but one could not deny how Witherspoon made the movie far more charming than it likely would have been with anyone else in the starring role. However, Blair also made a believable performance of a suspicious woman who eventually realized she was wrong. She may not have garnered as much attention and positive feedback as Witherspoon, but she did become a much more notable celebrity following this second successful movie.

The film remains popular today and has aged better than her first major role. Following the turn, as the romantic opponent turned friend, producers and directors were more interested in casting her. For the next decade, she would find herself fairly busy. Her next major project would become a cult classic, and her casting was likely thanks to the versatile Blair, who had proven to be in very different types of movies.

Chapter 6

Hellboy

In 2004, Blair managed to end up in another significant role in a very different type of movie. Where her first major role was in a dark teenage drama, and her second major role was in a teenage hit movie, her third major role was in a dark comic book movie, *Hellboy*. At the time, there had not been many successful comic book movies. By 2004, the few highly successful movies in this genre were Sam Raimi's *Spider-Man* (2002), *The Mask* (1994), some of the Christopher Reeve's *Superman* movies, Tim Burton's *Batman* (1989) and *Batman Returns* (1992), *Blade* (1998) and *Blade 2* (2002), and a handful of other movies. These movies were successful because they had recognizable characters, particularly *Spiderman*, *Superman*, and *Batman*. Before Marvel began churning out movies and shows regularly, committing to a comic book movie was a real risk, so movies in this genre were incredibly risky. The *Blade* movies and *Batman* movies were the only really successful dark comic book movies, making *Hellboy* a much riskier proposition for the studio. This is probably why they focused on casting people who could pull off the characters and make them likable. 2004 was also before the antihero boom, and with the lead character being an antihero – not a hero – this was a high-risk undertaking.

In part, Ron Perlman was cast in the titular character because of his unique appearance with a broader face and incredibly tall stature (6.0 tall, compared to the average height of 5 foot 9.5 inches for males in Hollywood). Selma Blair was cast as his love interest, a woman with a dark past. At about 5 foot 3 inches, Perlman had nearly a foot on her. Since he was already significantly taller than many of his co-stars, not as much was needed to be done to make him look significantly bigger. They were both ideal in their roles, and their very different looks helped to play into the aesthetics of the comic book characters.

Hellboy was the unintended result of Nazi experiments as they tried to make a demonic army to fight in World War II. Their attempt to create the army was thwarted by Trevor Bruttenhom, who finds the child created in the experiment. Initially calling the half-demon baby Hellboy, the name sticks, and the CIA brings up the child to the Bureau of Paranormal Research (BPRD). Liz Sherman (played by Blair) was a part of the BPRD because of her pyrokinetic abilities. She has committed herself to a mental hospital because she can no longer control her powers. The two grew up in the same facilities because of what they were; though she is human, she is a risk to those around her. Her backstory is that she accidentally killed her family because she could not control her abilities. There is chemistry between the characters at the beginning of the movie, but they are not yet romantically involved. This changes as Hellboy sees her going out for coffee with one of the other agents. Throughout the movie, they end up saving each other, and he finally makes it obvious that he is romantically interested in her at the end.

Though it is not a movie for everyone because of the darker elements, it was incredibly well-done for its time. Its critical success is largely because of the great casting. However, it was also directed by Guillermo del Toro, a director who has become an acclaimed director and screenwriter. It currently has an 81% Rotten Tomatoes score. It did well enough to get a sequel, though that did not receive another follow-up. The movies largely followed the comic books - Hellboy and Liz are just friends in the comic books, but the producers and studio probably felt that romance should be added to get more people to watch it. Because it largely stuck to the existing storyline, was visually stunning, was incredibly well cast, and had compelling plots, both movies continue to have a cult following today. It did well enough to eye the reboot treatment, though the 2019 movie did not meet the expectations of the first two films. One of the complaints was that people wanted to see the original cast and their progress in their lives, not rehash an earlier part of the story. The majority of fans were just as upset with the recasting of the titular character because Perlman seemed to embody the character so well in the first two movies. The fact that Del Toro was not directing also put fans off from going to see the reboot.

Again, Blair did not get much recognition from most fans, but they were eager to see her return to the role. They may not have seen her as embodying the character in quite the same way as the iconic Hellboy, but she did what she had done well in her previous works – she was a great supporting actor. When the reboot was announced instead of the third installment, she was open about being disappointed like the fans. However, she was politically savvy in that she expressed an interest in seeing how the new director and actors would do with the darker material. The original was PG-13, which meant it reached a younger fanbase than the R-rated reboot. The R rating was more appropriate for the material. However, fans still felt that Del Toro and Perlman would have done a fantastic job because they had already cleaned it up well enough to translate it for younger audiences. Fans may not be as verbally supportive of Blair, in large part because she seems to be a part of a package deal. Since she was instrumental in both films, it would be expected that she would reprise her role if the other two major players returned.

Chapter 7

Successful Career

Blair is one of the few actors easily identified by such a wide range of fanbases. Like Tim Curry, you can get an idea of what a person likes based on what they have seen Blair in. Not able to be typecast, she can mold into roles, playing what is needed and supporting the main cast. Besides these three roles, she also played Kate Wales, the therapist, in the TV show *Anger Management*. This is probably one of her other well-known parts. She has continued to play in dozens of other shows, including recurring characters and other movies. However, over time, she did seem to gravitate more toward indie films.

Around her 30th birthday, she started being considered for fewer roles focused more on the older, more mature women. She did manage to get another romantic leading role in *A Guy Thing*, and she talked openly about how waking up on her 30th birthday ended up being not much of an issue: "When that happened, I woke up the next morning and said: Oh my God, I can breathe." Given how many women have spoken about what happened to their career after hitting the 30th birthday milestone, this seemed to help destigmatize hitting the three-decade mark for women. While it was not quite the same as what happens at 40 years old, Blair had spent much of her early career playing teenagers and young adults, despite being well over those ages. She seemed to be following in the long line of women who wanted to make it known how they were treated after hitting a certain age, with the difference of adding some humor to it. At 30, many producers are looking to find younger women instead of those capable in their profession. Maggie Gyllenhaal has been one of the most recent women to speak out, saying that when she was 37 years old, she was told that she was "too old" to play the romantic partner for a man who was 55 years old. Based on an analysis of American films released between 1920 and 2011, when women reach 30 years old, they receive only 40% of leading roles. Perhaps the most eye-opening revelation came from one of the most well-respected actors of her generation, Meryl Streep. In 2015, she played the part of a witch in the musical *Into the Woods*. It was the first time that she had played a witch since turning 40 (she was 65 when she agreed to accept the part). During one interview, she told the reporter, "Our culture is pretty youth-obsessed, especially people that pass 40. I was not offered any female adventurers, love interests, or heroes, or demons. I was offered witches because I was 'old' at 40." She went on to say that she was offered three different witch roles the year that she reached her fourth decade. By that time, she had won three Oscars.

Blair started addressing the problem women face, particularly in Hollywood, as they age. While many women have expressed understandable anger, resentment, or frustration, Blair chose to go with humor to point out that nothing really changed. Crossing that artificial age line from 29 to 30 mainly was an issue she had built up in her head. It was not something she could stop or control.

Things have improved for women in entertainment, with bigger names being women in their 50s, like Nicole Kidman and Halle Berry. The changes are incremental, so the injection of humor into an emotional subject did help people to see it from a different perspective.

Blair went a little further in her discussion about aging, saying, "I don't' know what it was, but, before 30, I really felt I needed to please people…[now I want] to do everything, but I also have to be responsible to myself and need to have a little bit more control and power… The roles I have done for studio movies in the past have been very much supporting and character-driven, even if they are rather inconsequential roles, which I don't mind. I take every role very seriously and so I think maybe if you are just playing the foil to the beautiful, glamorous ones, it is bound to be the opposite of the beautiful glamorous one, and so you get me." The fact that she was able to laugh while discussing her more unique appearance highlights how she did not fit into the same mold as many other actors. She would need that sense of humor, though, as, toward the end of the 2010s, she would receive news that would entirely change her work prospects.

In 2016, she continued finding roles, including in *American Crime Story*, a TV series about high-profile crimes in the 1990s, including the OJ Simpson trial. In the series, she played Kris Jenner, wife to one of Simpson's lawyers at the trial. She also had a role on the TV show *Heathers* in 2018. None of her other work has landed quite like her early roles, but she was not concerned.

Chapter 8

Personal Life

Prior to 2018, Blair already had a lot of highs and lows that go beyond what most people experience. She was in a fairly high-profile relationship with Jason Schwartzman during the early part of the 2000s when she was gaining in popularity. She would later find out that one of her co-stars on the set of *Legally Blonde* had a crush on her, but she was already taken. Blair went on to marry Ahmed Zappa after dating for six months. They were able to wed at Carrier Fisher's home in 2004, and Blair has expressed how much she has always looked up to Fisher. She felt an affinity with the late actress because she also had a relatively rough life, though for very different reasons. Blair has pointed to a particular Fisher quote as being poignant to her; "If my life wasn't funny it would just be true, and that is unacceptable.".

The marriage only lasted about two years, with the couple's divorce being official in 2006. She dated several other notable men before becoming pregnant with her son. She did not marry her son's father, Jason Bleick, who is a fashion designer. They broke up a year after their son's birth.

With her son arriving in 2011, her priorities as a single mother began to shift. She once told *The Glow* that "I don't think any other miracle could have grounded me in this way – I appreciate every second I'm in his company." However, it wasn't until he was four years old that she finally gave up drinking. When she was traveling with her son and companion, Blair passed out on a plane because of a mix of prescription medications and alcohol. When she woke, she realized that she had to start making changes. She had tried to stop drinking on numerous occasions before that point, but she quickly found excuses to drink. She would say that as an alcoholic, she was high functioning, but she was not a social drinker because she knew that she could not control herself when she drank. She pointed out that being an alcoholic did not mean that she was always drunk. The problem was that she used drinking to cope or manage herself. Blair has been open about her struggles with depression, anxiety, and alcohol. However, she decided to stop when she realized just what was at stake and how negatively her drinking could affect her child. During an interview in 2022, she said that she still is an alcoholic because it is a life-long commitment not to drink. The difference is that now she does not allow herself to excuse drinking because it is "just this one," "just while on vacation," or any other excuses that she told herself to start drinking again.

Her son helped give her a reason to take better care of herself, but that also means that she feels the responsibility a lot more than she might otherwise feel it. Blair has highlighted that being a mom has similar problems no matter who you are, "As a mom, there's almost a shame in feeling too attached, like there's something shameful in saying, 'My kid is my life these days." There's a time and a place especially when they're this young. Let yourself enjoy it. I wish people would talk about love more." Some mothers feel guilted into spending less time with their children, while others feel guilted into spending more time with their children. Her point is that people express love differently, so they should be allowed to dote on their children or take breaks as needed. Blair also let other mothers know that she understood the problems of balancing a good mother with work. As a single mother, there is not as much choice, which has made her a lot more relatable to a wider audience.

One of the darkest chapters in her life occurred in 1999. Her agent sent her to a hotel room to meet with James Toback for a role. He told her that he would mentor her but said she had to prove that she trusted him. Allegedly, he said she had to do that by removing her clothing. She actually trusted her representative, thinking that her representative would not send her to someone who would do her harm. Unfortunately, this proved a bad assumption as Toback then reportedly sexually assaulted her. When he finished, he allegedly told her that he would have her killed if she told anyone. She would not say anything about it until 2017, after the *Me Too Movement* started toppling many high-profile men who preyed on women in similar positions. Nor was she the first to make allegations against him. She saw several accounts by women about similar experiences with the director, including Rachel McAdams. They all reported believing that they were safe, mainly as he kept telling them that he was pushing them out of their comfort zone to help them be better actors. This perhaps is true, but not the way he led them to believe it, as his alleged victims did not speak up for years after the abuse. Despite 38 women accusing him of sexual abuse, he never faced charges because of the statute of limitations. When asked, he said that all of the women were lying and then claimed that he had not met them or did not remember meeting them. Following Blair's account of what happened to her, the number of women who felt they could speak up significantly increased. As one of the most prominent women who leveled allegations against him, it helped others feel they could also speak up, which was her goal, especially after he tried to dismiss the allegations of others. Ultimately, it has been reported that more than 200 women have accused him of sexual assault or sexual harassment since that first account was published. Though it was difficult for her, Blair recounted, "I did think of my experience with James Toback and how shaming that was and how angry I was to have to be silent for so long because I was afraid. … just being free of the shame was huge." However, it is a part of her past that she has not wanted to relive. She prefers to leave it in the past to focus on what is important to her now.

In February 2022, she wound up in the hospital, and she made allegations against her boyfriend that he had attacked her. It was another horrible event in her life, but one that she is eager to put behind her. She successfully got a restraining order against him, and he tried to get one against her, though the court denied his filing. When discussing the event, she expressed the idea that it was surreal, and she had a hard time believing that it was happening. During a 2022 interview, Blair confided, "I feel much more secure in my life. As long as my son is okay, and I don't have an immediate death sentence or am in immediate peril, then I could probably handle anything."

Chapter 9

Multiple Sclerosis

If 2017 was a big year because she finally spoke out, accusing Tobeck of sexual assault, 2018 was difficult for a new reason. Blair had suffered from a number of health issues over the years, but nothing seemed to be helping much. She was two years into being sober, so the problem clearly was not alcohol. In the latter half of 2018, she went to the doctor believing she was suffering from a pinched nerve. She was trying to identify where she fell over in front of her doctor. He realized that the problem was more severe than a pinched nerve. She was soon diagnosed with multiple sclerosis (MS).

According to the Mayo Clinic, MS is a "potentially disabling disease of the brain and spinal cord." It can present as early as childhood, and scans have been done to check children's spines to ensure they are not showing early signs. It is a degenerative disease, so it will continue to worsen over time. The question is:

How much of the steady decline can be avoided or minimized? There is no cure for MS.

When she learned that she had the disease and what it was, Blair took some time to process what it meant. She then went online to announce what she had learned. Since it is not a disease that is often discussed, there aren't many people who speak out about having it and what it is like to deal with the problems it causes. Blair pointed out that she had probably been suffering from it for at least 15 years by the time she was diagnosed because people had not considered her symptoms to be an indication of MS. What was even more disheartening was that her MS had been worse following the birth of her son, which was why she had been feeling so much worse. She had suffered postpartum depression, but that could probably have been lessened had she been diagnosed earlier with MS. Drinking had helped her to cope until she finally gave that up too. That meant that she was in almost perpetual pain.

Some diagnoses bring a heavy burden, but for Blair, actually getting diagnosed with something was a huge relief. Something had been wrong for years, but she had not realized that it was something much worse than the minor ailments that she and her doctors had been trying to treat. Until she was diagnosed, she felt that the problem was her, and it had led to her trying to act like she was okay, even though she wanted her doctors to help her fix the problem. The shame and guilt that she felt about not being able to talk about the problem finally subsided when they figured out what was wrong with her, and why she couldn't seem to get rid of the pain. More importantly, she could finally start looking for a more effective treatment.

She acknowledged that it was painful and that she lost a lot for a while because of MS. However, she wanted to make sure that she knew better than to sit around feeling sorry for herself. During an interview with Vanity Fair, she said, "I do not feel sorry for myself in life. At all. I believe in unraveling the necklace to make it useful again. And sometimes, the knots are tight and difficult to undo. So we must be gentle with our traumas." Over time, she would time to realize that she was far from the only person who tried to hide her pain and suffering. In the same interview, she admitted, "when I read comments on Instagram form people who were suffering, whether it was form MS, or anything, I thought, holy shit, there's a need for honesty about being disabled from someone recognizable."

Blair has been very open about her problems, letting people watch her through some of the worst of what she has dealt with following the diagnosis. In 2019, she made her first red carpet appearance since she had let the world know about her condition. She was invited to the Vanity Fair Oscars party, and she showed up in a flowing gown with black and pastels. A chocker-like necklace wrapped around her neck, highlighting the flowing cap-like aspect of the gown that seemed to flow from it. She looked stunning, but she had an accessory that no other celebrity had: a custom-designed cane to help her walk. She said that she was interested in working with a designer to make more fashion that was more friendly for people with disabilities. In her own words, "You shouldn't have to sacrifice style." Her look at the time made it clear that there was a lot to explore in terms of fashion for the disabled. She received much attention for her elegant look that was somewhat reminiscent of earlier ages when people carried canes as much as a fashion statement as a physical need.

In 2021, she was the subject of a documentary about living with MS. *Introducing, Selma Blair* was released in 2021, and it revealed the celebrity's struggle with her body's decline. As someone who has said that she is more shy than outgoing, Blair found talking to people to be helpful through the pain. The documentary was meant to show the messier side that people tend to want to ignore or that makes them feel shame or vulnerability. She had elected to undergo a stem-cell transplant back in 2019, which was included in the documentary. Following the procedure, patients undergo chemotherapy, resulting in hair loss. As she had expressed earlier, she wanted anyone who felt challenged or unsure to find some inspiration or familiarity, even if they were suffering from something other than a chronic ailment. She put it best when she said, "This is my human condition and everyone has their own, but I think we are united in feeling alone or frightened when we have a big change in our lives. This wasn't a vanity project at all, and I'm very capable of loving vanity." It was also to help her better understand herself as she can see where she was before the treatment and how she has progressed since. Blair said that being older helped her do the documentary because she didn't feel ashamed of her condition. Most of the problems that she had experienced from childhood, the reason she had started drinking so young, were likely linked to MS. She had suffered mood swings, aches, fatigue, and pain most of her life. It only got worse as she aged, to the point where she was losing eyesight after her son was born. Then there were muscle contractions in her neck. The documentary shows the kinds of symptoms she had over the course of filming, even after treatment. It also was a much more honest look as Blair did not hold any control over the editing of the project. Staying true to her word, she wanted it to be more like a diary that showed her struggles.

She did survive, and has even watched the first 20 minutes with her son. At that point, he was too uncomfortable with it, fearing that it might prevent her from getting acting jobs or causing people to gossip about her. Blair has said she still wants to work as an actress, but most of her roles are for disabled people in wheelchairs. Just like she did not want her age to define her when she was young, she wants people to know that she has not changed since the diagnosis. She just knows what is wrong now. However, she continues to talk about her experiences to help other people, even if it does hamper her career because that seems to be more important to her.

Besides, she does have other outlets, as she proved in the early part of 2022. She is now able to walk her dog and do things more like she used to because her MS was in remission.

Chapter 10

A Cathartic Memoir

Blair has said that people have told her that she should write about her experiences, but she was reluctant. While there were a lot of inspirational aspects of her life, there was a lot of misery and pain that she had used alcohol to manage. She earned a degree in English, so she knew how to work with the language, but that isn't the same thing as actually reliving painful experiences for others to read. Being filmed for a documentary was painful at the moment; writing a book of memoirs was going back and reliving all of the pain over a life full of extreme highs and lows for her. However, it offered her a chance to look back over her life and understand how MS had affected her over her life. Some of the erratic behavior, the unexplained pain, and emotions were painful to revisit, but they would make more sense if she were willing to go back through her life to see how MS had likely affected her since she was young.

Around the time she started her book, Blair's mother died. It gave the actress another angle for the tale she needed to tell as she had now lost the formidable woman who had raised her to be formidable herself. The loss also seemed to help spur her on to finish the book.

The full title of her memoir is *Mean Baby: A Memoir of Growing Up*. It is an interesting title, and it comes from the way people characterized her personality when she was an infant. People would tell her that "she was a mean, mean baby." The book is an entertaining and candid look at a life with an inordinate number of highs and lows that seems unreal to most people.

Conclusion

Selma Blair's life thus far has been unpredictable and inspiring. Her early interest in writing would take decades to manifest in a book, yet her belief that a girl from Michigan could make it as an actress led her to relative fame. MS has been in the background most of her life, affecting her in ways she didn't know until she was diagnosed in 2018. Despite having the disease, she was able to make a name for herself in one of the most notoriously difficult industries. She was happy with being a supporting character, earning her a much wider range of characters in various genres. As she aged, she became more open about her experiences, apparently starting with being an "aging actress" on her 30th birthday and struggling with depression and anxiety. Over time, she turned to even more complicated subjects, including the sexual abuse in the industry. When she was diagnosed with MS, Blair did not hesitate to be open about it and let people see just what it was like to live with an incurable disease. Not only has she amassed a wealth of fans because of her diverse characters, but she has earned an entirely new fanbase of people who appreciate or are inspired by her struggles.

Made in the USA
Las Vegas, NV
06 July 2022